THE *Skinny*
SPIRALIZER
RECIPE BOOK

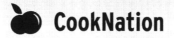

THE SKINNY SPIRALIZER RECIPE BOOK

Delicious Spiralizer Inspired Low Calorie Recipes For One. All Under 200, 300, 400 & 500 Calories

Copyright © Bell & Mackenzie Publishing Limited 2014

ISBN 978-1-909855-70-0

A CIP catalogue record of this book is available from the British Library

• •

DISCLAIMER

This book is designed to provide information on meals, sides and snacks that can be made in conjunction with a tri-blade spiralizer vegetable device. Results may differ if alternative devices are used.

Some recipes may contain nuts or traces of nuts. Those suffering from any allergies associated with nuts should avoid any recipes containing nuts or nut based oils.

This information is provided and sold with the knowledge that the publisher and author do not offer any legal or other professional advice.

In the case of a need for any such expertise consult with the appropriate professional.

This book does not contain all information available on the subject, and other sources of recipes are available.

This book has not been created to be specific to any individual's requirements.

Every effort has been made to make this book as accurate as possible. However, there may be typographical and or content errors. Therefore, this book should serve only as a general guide and not as the ultimate source of subject information.

This book contains information that might be dated and is intended only to educate and entertain.

The author and publisher shall have no liability or responsibility to any person or entity regarding any loss or damage incurred, or alleged to have incurred, directly or indirectly, by the information contained in this book.

CONTENTS

UNDER 400 CALORIES

UNDER 500 CALORIES

CONVERSION CHART

OTHER COOKNATION TITLES

INTRODUCTION

If you are looking for new and fresh meal ideas to use with your spiralizer then this book is for you.

Welcome to The Skinny Spiralizer Recipe Book. Here you will discover delicious, healthy, low calorie, low carb complete meals-for-one taking inspiration from your vegetable spiralizer. All our recipes make creative and nutritious meals using meat, fish and vegetables as well as some hearty soups and tasty salads. We love vegetables but this isn't a vegetarian cookbook!

If you are looking for new and fresh meal ideas to use with your spiralizer then this book is for you.

The spiralizer is the ideal companion for anyone who may be following a diet, is cutting down on their carbohydrates or just wants to increase their vegetable intake in an inspirational way. The spiralizer can help you shed pounds as part of a balanced calorie controlled diet, turning vegetables into guilt-free squash 'pasta', sweet potato 'rice', zucchini 'noodles', cucumber ribbons, carrot spirals and more.

The spiralizer has taken the US by storm and it's about to do the same in the UK, bringing with it a multitude of tasty recipe opportunities. Followers of popular diets such as the 5:2 Fast Diet, Paleo Diet and Atkins Diet will find the spiralizer their most used kitchen appliance. Plus, if you have a young family the spiralizer is a fantastic way of engaging young children with vegetables making them fun, interesting and tasty!

HOW DOES IT WORK? In its most basic form, a spiralizer turns vegetables into noodles – a godsend for anyone who loves pasta – but can also create veggie spaghetti, ribbons, spirals and more making vegetables at mealtimes an art form. It is a manual gadget that requires no electricity. Gripping a vegetable like a vice and cranking the handle pushes the vegetable through a sharp blade to create vegetable spirals. Once spiralized, you are left with the central core of the vegetable which can either be discarded or chopped up and used in your recipe.

The most popular spiralizer devices come with 3 interchangeable blades. The names of these blades may differ depending on which device you own but they will all deliver similar results.

Shredder Blade – creates thin spaghetti-like noodles
Chipper Blade – creates thicker noodles
Straight/Slicer Blade – creates ribbons/slices

The blades are very sharp and care should be taken when handling and cleaning them. It helps to use a knife to remove any leftover vegetable from the blades before washing.

The spiralizer comes with rubber suction cups on the base that provide much needed stability when applying pressure to turn the handle. Push the device down firmly on your counter top to prevent sliding and have a bowl/plate/chopping board in place to catch the spirals.

Cleaning your spiralizer couldn't be easier. It should come apart into 3 main components: the base, the handle and the blade. Everything except the metal blade is made of plastic which can be easily washed or placed in the dishwasher (blades included). Just make sure you rinse everything under the tap first to remove any leftover vegetables.

There are a number of vegetables that work particularly well with the spiralizer. Some won't work so well. Generally speaking vegetables that are hollow, are too small or don't have a solid shape are not suitable for spiralizing. The following are the vegetables used most commonly in our recipes but this is by no means an extensive list and experimenting by yourself is all part of the fun! Remember that while there are plenty of vegetables that may not be suitable for spiralizing, they can still be cooked and added to your plate. Most of our recipes use a wide range of veg to make up your meal.

Courgette/Zucchini
Sweet Potatoes
Cucumber
Carrot
Beetroot
Aubergine/Eggplant
Apple
Cucumber
Butternut Squash

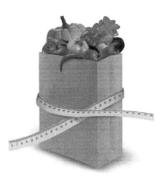

When shopping for your vegetables try to choose larger, fatter varieties as they give much better results.

The spiralized vegetables in our recipes range from being eaten raw, blanched in boiling water, oven baked, boiled and stir-fried. As the emphasis of this recipe book is healthy, low calorie meals it's important to remember not to use excessive amounts of cooking oil that can be high in saturated fats and calories. Make sure you have to hand a good quality extra virgin olive oil and low calorie cooking oil spray. Only a small amount is needed to cook evenly. Using good quality non-stick pans will also reduce the need for excessive oil.

OUR SKINNY RECIPES

All our recipes are simple and easy to follow and all fall below 200, 300, 400 or 500 calories each. Many use low calorie and low fat alternatives to everyday products. We would encourage you to add these to your shopping basket each week and make a point of paying attention to food labelling whenever you can - some low fat products can be very high in sugar so watch out! Try switching to some of the following everyday items to keep calories and fat lower and be sure to take note of our kitchen essentials.

Low fat yogurt
Semi skimmed/half fat milk
Reduced fat cheese
Low fat/unsaturated 'butter' spreads
Low cal cooking oil spray
Low fat cream/half and half

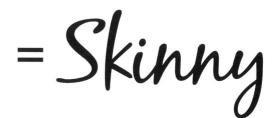

STORE CUPBOARD ESSENTIALS

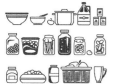

All our skinny low calorie recipes use simple, easily obtainable, store cupboard ingredients. To maintain a healthy diet we recommend keeping your kitchen stocked up with many of the following essentials and plenty of fresh fruit, veg & lean meat too!

Turmeric
Dijon mustard
Honey
Dried Italian herbs
Olive oil
Balsamic vinegar
Soy Sauce
Papirka
Free range eggs
Crushed sea salt
Worcestershire/A1 steak sauce
Tinned/Canned tuna
Tinned/canned chopped tomatoes
Ground black pepper
Thai fish sauce

Tomato puree/paste
Tomato passata/sauce
Mixed tinned/canned beans
Lemon juice
Lime juice
Cider Vinegar
Rice wine vinegar
Pitted black olives
Chicken & vegetable stock
Crushed chilli flakes
Dried fruit & nuts
Fresh Garlic
Fresh ginger
Ground coriander/cilantro

WEIGHT MANAGEMENT TIPS

If you are spiralizing to manage your weight or following a diet, we've put together some helpful tips to help you avoid some of the most common pitfalls. Any change of diet requires willpower and motivation but half the battle is knowing what to expect so you can better prepare yourself to achieve your goals.

• Eat slowly. There's no rush. Eating very quickly is no good for your digestive system and chances are you'll be looking for second helpings before your body has even had the chance to feel satisfied.

• Chew. It sounds obvious but you should properly chew your food and swallow only when it's broken down and you have enjoyed what you have tasted.

• Wait. Before reaching for second helpings wait 5-10 minutes and let your body tell you whether you are still hungry. More often than not, the answer will be no and you will be satisfied with the meal you have had. A glass of water before each meal will help you with any cravings for more. Remember you are on a fast day and restricting your calories. Be realistic about what to expect.

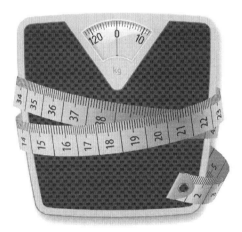

• Avoid too much exercise at first. If you have just started a diet, eating less is likely to make you feel a little weaker, certainly to start with, so don't put the pressure on yourself to work out initially.

• Avoid alcohol. Not only is alcohol packed with calories it could also have a greater effect on you than usual if you are on a diet.

• Drink plenty of water throughout the day. Water is your best friend. It's good for you, has zero calories, and will fill you up & help stop you feeling hungry. Have a glass before and also with your meal.

• When you are eating each meal, put your fork down between bites – it will make you eat more slowly and you'll feel fuller on less food.

• Brush your teeth immediately after your meal to discourage yourself from eating more.

• If you get food cravings (and you will), acknowledge them, and then distract yourself. Go out for a walk, phone a friend or play with the kids.

• Whenever hunger hits, try waiting 15 minutes and ride out the cravings. You'll find they pass and you can move on with your day.

• Remember - feeling hungry is not a bad thing. The norm is to act on the smallest hunger pangs - we've forgotten what it's like to feel genuinely hungry. Learn to 'own' your hunger and take control of how you deal with it.

• Get moving. As with all diets, increased activity will complement your weight loss efforts. Think about what you are doing each day: choose the stairs instead of the lift, walk to the shops instead of driving. Making small changes will not only help you burn calories but will make you feel healthier and more in control of your weight loss.

• Stay motivated. Think about what you are trying to achieve and stick with it. Keep your eye on the prize. If you have a bad day forget about it, don't feel guilty. Recognise where you went wrong and move on. Tomorrow is a new day!

ABOUT COOKNATION

CookNation is the leading publisher of innovative and practical recipe books for the modern, health conscious cook.

CookNation titles bring together delicious, easy and practical recipes with their unique approach - easy and delicious, no-nonsense recipes - making cooking for diets and healthy eating fast, simple and fun.

With a range of #1 best-selling titles - from the innovative 'Skinny' calorie-counted series, to the 5:2 Diet Recipes collection - CookNation recipe books prove that 'Diet' can still mean 'Delicious'!

Turn to the end of this book to browse all CookNation's recipe books

www.cooknationbooks.com
www.bellmackenzie.com

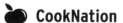 CookNation

THE *Skinny* SPIRALIZER

UNDER 200 CALORIES

LEMONGRASS & SHRIMP CLEAR BROTH

175 calories per serving

Ingredients

- 1 courgette/zucchini weighing 200g/7oz
- 1 tsp olive oil
- 75g/3oz raw, shelled king prawns/jumbo shrimp
- ½ lemongrass stalk, finely chopped
- ½ red chilli, deseeded & finely sliced
- ½ onion, sliced
- 1 tsp freshly grated ginger
- 1 garlic clove, crushed
- 2 tsp soy sauce
- 370ml/1½ cups chicken stock
- 2 tbsp lime juice
- Salt & pepper to taste

Method

1 Top & tail the courgette and use the shredder blade to turn into thin noodles.

2 Gently heat a non-stick saucepan on the hob with the olive oil and sauté the prawns, lemongrass, chilli, onion, ginger & garlic for 2 minutes.

3 Add the soy sauce, stock & courgette noodles and simmer for 3-5 minutes or until the noodles are tender and the prawns are cooked through.

4 Stir through the lime juice, season and serve.

CHEFS NOTE
Half a teaspoon of ground ginger is fine to use if you don't have fresh root ginger.

SESAME & SUGAR SNAP SOUP

150 calories per serving

Ingredients

- 1 courgette/zucchini weighing 200g/7oz
- 1 tsp sesame oil
- ½ onion, sliced
- 1 garlic clove, crushed
- ½ tsp freshly grated ginger
- 75g/3oz sugar snap peas
- ½ pak choi/bok choi, shredded
- A pinch of crushed chilli flakes
- 2 tsp soy sauce
- 370ml/1½ cups chicken stock
- Salt & pepper to taste

Method

1 Top & tail the courgette and use the shredder blade to turn into thin noodles.

2 Gently heat a non-stick saucepan on the hob with the olive oil and sauté the onion, ginger & garlic for 2 minutes.

3 Add the peas, pak choi, chilli flakes, soy sauce, stock & courgette noodles and simmer for 3-5 minutes or until the noodles are tender.

4 Season and serve.

CHEFS NOTE

If you don't have pak choi use shredded pointed cabbage.

FRESH LIME ZUCCHINI RIBBONS

195
calories per serving

Ingredients

- Courgettes/Zucchini weighing 300g/11oz
- 1 tbsp olive oil
- ½ red chilli, deseeded & finely chopped
- Zest & juice of ½ lime
- 1 tsp honey
- Large pinch of sea salt
- Salt & pepper to taste

Method

1 Top & tail the courgettes and use the slicer/straight blade to turn into ribbons.

2 Place the ribbons in a bowl with the olive oil, chilli, lime juice, zest, honey and salt.

3 Combine really well to coat every inch of the courgette in the olive oil.

4 Leave to marinade for a few minutes and serve.

CHEFS NOTE
Eat as a light lunch or serve as a side to grilled fish or chicken.

BEETROOT & YOGURT SOUP

120 calories per serving

Ingredients

- 200g/7oz beetroot
- 1 tsp olive oil
- ½ onion, sliced
- 1 garlic clove, crushed
- 250ml/1 cup vegetable or chicken stock
- 1 tbsp fat free Greek yogurt
- Salt & pepper to taste

Method

1 Peel the beetroot and use the shredder blade to turn into thin spirals.

2 Take a knife and, holding the spirals in bunches, roughly chop into 1cm/½ inch pieces.

3 Gently heat a non-stick saucepan on the hob with the olive oil and sauté the sliced onion & garlic for a few minutes until softened.

4 Add the stock and beetroot to the pan and simmer for 5 minutes or until the beetroot is tender and the soup is piping hot.

5 Season and serve with a dollop of yogurt in the centre.

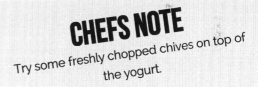

CHEFS NOTE
Try some freshly chopped chives on top of the yogurt.

CREAM CHEESE COLESLAW

130 calories per serving

Ingredients

- Carrots weighing 300g/11oz
- 1 apple
- 1 beetroot 75g/3oz
- 1 tbsp sultanas, finely chopped
- 1 tbsp low fat cream cheese

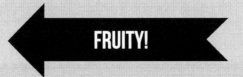

FRUITY!

Method

1 Top, tail & peel the carrots. Peel & core the apple. Peel the beetroot.

2 Use the shredder blade to turn the carrots, apple & beetroot into thin spirals.

3 Combine everything together really well in a bowl. Cover and chill in the fridge.

CHEFS NOTE
Use as a side for chicken or as a crudité dip.

GARLIC CHICKEN & CUCUMBER RIBBONS

195 calories per serving

Ingredients

- 1 cucumber
- 1 tsp sea salt
- 125g/4oz chicken breast, sliced
- 2 garlic cloves, crushed
- 1 tbsp soy sauce
- Pinch of crushed chillies
- Low cal cooking oil Spray
- Salt & pepper to taste

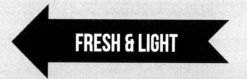

FRESH & LIGHT

Method

1 Top & tail the cucumber and use the straight/slicer blade to turn into thin ribbons.

2 Sprinkle with sea salt and set to one side in a colander where it will drain. Leave for 15 minutes, rinse through with cold water and thoroughly dry off.

3 Gently heat a large non-stick frying pan on the hob with a little low cal oil.

4 Add the sliced chicken & garlic and cook for 3 minutes. Add the soy sauce and chillies and cook for a further minute.

5 Add the cucumber ribbons, stir-fry for three minutes, season and serve.

CHEFS NOTE

This is a really simple little lunch. Serve with spiralized carrots if you want to bulk it up a little.

MOROCCAN CARROT RELISH

195
calories per serving

Ingredients

- Carrots weighing 300g/11oz
- 1 orange
- 2 pitted dates, finely chopped
- 1 tbsp sultanas, finely chopped
- ½ tsp brown sugar
- Small pinch of cinnamon (optional)

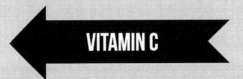

VITAMIN C

Method

1 Top, tail & peel the carrots and use the shredder blade to turn into thin spirals.

2 Peel the orange, divide into segments and finely chop.

3 Combine everything together really well in a bowl. Cover and chill in the fridge.

CHEFS NOTE
Use as a salad side or as a relish for meat dishes.

HONEY & THYME EGGPLANT

160 calories per serving

Ingredients

- 1 aubergine/egg plant weighing 300g/11oz
- 1 tsp olive oil
- Large pinch of dried thyme
- Large pinch of sea salt

- 1 tsp honey
- Twist of lemon juice
- 50g/2oz watercress or rocket
- Salt & pepper to taste

Method

1 Top & tail the aubergine and use the slicer/straight blade to turn into ribbons.

2 Gently heat the oil in a large non-stick frying pan on the hob. Add the ribbons, thyme, salt and honey to the pan. Combine well and cook for 4-6 minutes or until the aubergines are cooked though.

3 Stir through the lemon juice and tip onto a bed of watercress to serve.

CHEFS NOTE

This makes a simple supper for one or a veggie side dish for two.

CITRUS & BASIL ZUCCHINI SALAD

190 calories per serving

Ingredients

- Courgettes/Zucchini weighing 300g/11oz
- Zest & juice of ½ lemon
- 1 tbsp olive oil
- Pinch of salt
- 2 spring onions/scallions, finely sliced lengthways
- 1 tbsp freshly chopped basil
- Salt & pepper to taste

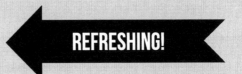

REFRESHING!

Method

1 Top & tail the courgettes and use the slicer/ straight blade to turn into ribbons.

2 In a bowl mix together the zest, lemon juice, olive oil & salt.

3 Add the ribbons to the bowl and toss together so that everything is coated with the oil and lemon.

4 Pile onto a plate and sprinkle over the sliced spring onion and chopped basil.

CHEFS NOTE
Season with plenty of freshly ground black pepper.

ONION & BALSAMIC DRESSED 'PASTA'

130
calories per serving

Ingredients

- Courgettes/Zucchini weighing 300g/11oz
- 1 tsp olive oil
- 1 garlic clove, crushed
- ½ red onion, chopped
- 2 sundried tomatoes, finely chopped
- 2 tbsp balsamic vinegar
- Salt & pepper to taste

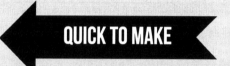

QUICK TO MAKE

Method

1 Top & tail the courgettes and use the shredder blade to turn into spaghetti noodles.

2 Gently heat a large non-stick frying pan on the hob with the olive oil.

3 Add the garlic, red onion, sundried tomatoes & balsamic vinegar and sauté for a few minutes until softened.

4 Add the spaghetti noodles and move around the pan for 3-5 minutes or until everything is piping hot.

5 Season and serve.

CHEFS NOTE

This simple dish also makes a good 'side' to pan-fried Tuna steaks.

SPIRALIZED BUBBLE & SQUEAK

190 calories per serving

Ingredients

- 1 sweet potato weighing 125g/4oz
- 1 courgette/zucchini weighing 200g/7oz
- ½ onion, sliced
- 1 garlic clove, crushed
- 1 tsp medium curry powder
- 1 tbsp water
- Low cal cooking oil spray
- Salt & pepper to taste

Method

1 Peel the sweet potato and use the chipper blade to turn into thick spirals.

2 Top & tail the courgette and use the shredder blade to turn into thin noodles.

3 Cook the potato spirals in salted boiling water for 2-3 minutes. Drain and put to one side.

4 Gently heat a large non-stick frying pan on the hob with a little low cal spray, add the onions & garlic and cook for a few minutes until softened.

5 Mix together the curry powder and water and add this to the pan along with the sweet potato spirals and courgettes noodles.

6 Increase the heat a little, combine well and cook for about 5-7 minutes or until everything is golden brown and piping hot (add a splash of water to the pan if you need to loosen it up).

7 Check the seasoning and serve.

CHEFS NOTE
Try breaking an egg into the pan and binding everything together into a hash.

SUNDRIED TOMATO & BASIL 'PASTA'

195 calories per serving

Ingredients

- 1 large courgette/zucchini, weighing 300g/11oz
- ½ onion, chopped
- 1 garlic clove, crushed
- 200g/7oz vine ripened tomatoes, chopped
- 1 tbsp sundried tomato puree/paste
- 1 tbsp freshly chopped basil
- ½ tsp each salt & brown sugar
- 1 tbsp low fat cream/half & half
- Low cal cooking oil spray
- Salt & pepper to taste

Method

1 Top & tail the courgette and use the shredder blade to turn into spaghetti noodles.

2 Heat a large non-stick frying pan on the hob with a little low cal spray.

3 Gently sauté the onions, garlic, tomatoes, puree, basil, salt & sugar for 8-10 minutes or until the tomatoes are cooked through.

4 Tip the contents of the pan into a blender and pulse until you have a smooth sauce. Add a little water or some stock to alter the consistency if you wish.

5 Add the spaghetti noodles to the empty frying pan and move around the pan for 3-5 minutes or until they are piping hot.

6 Tip the noodles into a bowl, pour over the tomato sauce. Season and serve.

CHEFS NOTE
Garnish with chopped fresh basil leaves.

MARINATED COURGETTE RIBBONS

190 calories per serving

Ingredients

- Courgettes/Zucchini weighing 300g/11oz
- 1 tbsp olive oil
- 1 garlic clove, crushed
- Zest & juice of ½ lemon
- Large pinch of sea salt
- 1 tbsp freshly chopped basil
- Salt & pepper to taste

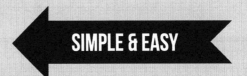

SIMPLE & EASY

Method

1 Top & tail the courgettes and use the straight/slicer blade to turn into ribbons.

2 Place the ribbons in a bowl with the olive oil, garlic, lemon juice & zest. Combine really well to coat every inch of the courgette in the olive oil.

3 Gently heat a large non-stick frying pan on the hob and add the ribbons to the pan. Cook for a couple of minutes and plate up.

4 Sprinkle with the sea salt and chopped basil to serve.

CHEFS NOTE

This is even better if you leave it to marinate for an hour or two before eating as a chilled dish.

CREAMY SQUASH SAUCE 'SPAGHETTI'

195 calories per serving

Ingredients

- Courgettes/Zucchini weighing 300g/11oz
- 150g/5oz butternut squash flesh, peeled, deseeded & finely chopped
- 2 tsp freshly chopped sage
- ½ onion, chopped
- 1 garlic clove, crushed
- 60ml/¼ cup hot vegetable stock
- 2 tbsp low fat cream
- Low cal cooking oil spray
- Salt & pepper to taste

Method

1 Top & tail the courgettes and use the shredder blade to turn into spaghetti noodles.

2 Heat a large non-stick frying pan on the hob with a little low cal spray and gently sauté the squash, sage, onion & garlic for about 8-10 minutes or until it's softened and cooked through (add a dash of water to the pan if you need to loosen it up).

3 When the squash and onions are ready place in a blender along with the hot stock. Pulse until you have a smooth sauce and add a little more water or stock to alter the consistency if you need to.

4 Add the spaghetti noodles to the empty frying pan and move around the pan for 3-5 minutes or until they are piping hot.

5 Add the squash sauce combine well, season and serve.

CHEFS NOTE
Dried sage is also fine to use for this simple pasta sauce recipe.

GARLIC & BROCCOLI 'PASTA'

195 calories per serving

Ingredients

- Courgettes/Zucchini weighing 300g/11oz
- 2 tsp olive oil
- 2 garlic cloves, crushed
- 150g/5oz purple sprouting broccoli/ Broccolini, finely chopped
- ½ onion, chopped
- 1 tsp anchovy paste
- Salt & pepper to taste

Method

1 Top & tail the courgettes and use the shredder blade to turn into spaghetti noodles.

2 Gently heat a large non-stick frying pan on the hob with the olive oil. Sauté the garlic, chopped broccoli, onions and anchovy paste for a few minutes until softened (add a splash of water to the pan if it needs loosening up).

3 Add the spaghetti noodles and move around the pan for 3-5 minutes or until everything is piping hot.

4 Season and serve.

CHEFS NOTE

Any type of young tenderstem broccoli works well for this recipe, sauté for longer if you prefer the broccoli soft.

THE *Skinny*
SPIRALIZER

UNDER 300 CALORIES

GRILLED COD ON A BED OF SPIRALS

270 calories per serving

Ingredients

- 1 courgette/zucchini weighing 200g/11oz
- 1 carrot weighing 200g/11oz
- 150g/5oz skinless, boneless cod loin
- Zest & juice of ¼ lemon
- 1 tbsp low fat 'butter' spread
- Low cal cooking oil spray
- Salt & pepper to taste

Method

1 Preheat the grill to a medium/high heat.

2 Top & tail the courgette, peel the carrot and use the shredder blade to turn into thin spirals.

3 Season the cod, spray with a little low cal oil and brush with the zest and lemon juice.

4 Place under the preheated grill and, turning once, cook for 8-10 minutes or until the fish is cooked through.

5 Meanwhile gently heat the 'butter' in a non-stick frying pan. Add the courgette and carrot spirals and cook for 3-4 minutes or until tender.

6 Arrange the cooked vegetables on a plate, sit the grilled cod on top. Season and serve.

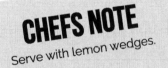

CHEFS NOTE
Serve with lemon wedges.

CHICKEN MISO SOUP

215
calories per serving

Ingredients

- 1 courgette/zucchini weighing 200g/7oz
- 1 tsp olive oil
- 75g/3oz chicken breast, thinly sliced
- 1 stalk celery, chopped
- ½ onion, sliced

- 1 garlic clove, crushed
- 2 tsp soy sauce
- 2 tsp miso paste
- 370ml/1½ cups boiling water
- Salt & pepper to taste

Method

1 Top & tail the courgette and use the shredder blade to turn into thin noodles.

2 Gently heat a non-stick saucepan on the hob with the olive oil and sauté the sliced chicken, celery, onion & garlic for 4 minutes.

3 Add the soy sauce, miso paste, water & courgette noodles and simmer for 3-5 minutes or until the noodles are tender and the chicken is cooked through.

4 Season and serve.

CHEFS NOTE

Add extra miso paste if you prefer a more intense flavour.

SWEET POTATO & SUNDRIED TOMATO SAUCE

250 calories per serving

Ingredients

- 1 large sweet potato weighing 200g/7oz
- 2 tbsp pitted black olives, sliced
- 2 tsp olive oil
- ½ onion, sliced
- ½ tsp dried oregano
- 1 tbsp sundried tomato puree/paste
- A pinch of crushed chilli flakes
- Salt & pepper to taste

Method

1 Peel the sweet potato and use the shredder blade to turn into spiralized sweet potato spaghetti.

2 Cook the spirals in salted boiling water for 1-1 ½ minutes. Drain and put to one side.

3 Gently heat a large non-stick frying pan on the hob with the olive oil and sauté the onions and oregano for a few minutes until softened. Stir through the sundried tomato puree and add the sweet potato spaghetti and chilli flakes.

4 Move about the pan for a couple of minutes until everything is piping hot (add a splash of water to the pan if you need to loosen it up).

5 Season and serve.

CHEFS NOTE
You could also try including a teaspoon of chopped capers when you sauté the onions.

WOK EGG SOUP

210
calories per serving

Ingredients

- 1 courgette/zucchini weighing 150g/5oz
- 1 garlic clove, crushed
- 1 tsp grated ginger
- ½ onion, sliced
- 75g/3oz mushrooms, sliced
- 1 tsp olive oil
- 1 tbsp soy sauce
- 370ml/1½ cups vegetable stock
- 1 free range egg
- Salt & pepper to taste

Method

1 Top & tail the courgette and use the shredder blade to turn into thin noodles.

2 Gently heat a wok on the hob with the olive oil and sauté the garlic, ginger, onion & mushrooms for a few minutes until softened.

3 Add the soy sauce & stock and simmer for a minute or two.

4 Beat the egg in a cup and, whilst stirring the soup, slowly pour the egg into the wok so that it sets into long 'strands'.

5 Add the courgette noodles and gently simmer for approx. 3 minutes or until tender.

6 Check the seasoning and serve in a shallow bowl.

CHEFS NOTE
Garnish with some chopped spring onions and chillies if you like.

BEEF 'NOODLE' SOUP

270 calories per serving

Ingredients

- 1 courgette/zucchini weighing 150g/5oz
- 1 tsp olive oil
- 75g/3oz steak, sliced
- 1 garlic clove, crushed
- ½ onion, sliced
- 75g/3oz mushrooms, sliced
- 75g/3oz green beans, chopped
- 370ml/1½ cups chicken stock
- 6 spring onions/scallions, finely chopped
- Low cal cooking oil spray
- Salt & pepper to taste

Method

1 Top & tail the courgette and use the shredder blade to turn into thin noodles.

2 Gently heat a non-stick saucepan on the hob with the olive oil and sauté the steak, garlic, onion, mushrooms & green beans for 2 minutes.

3 Add the stock and courgette noodles and simmer for approx. 3 minutes or until the noodles are tender and the steak is cooked through.

4 Serve in a shallow bowl with the spring onions over the top.

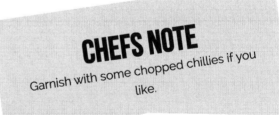

CHEFS NOTE
Garnish with some chopped chillies if you like.

CURRIED TOMATO & SWEET POTATO SOUP

295
calories per serving

Ingredients

- 1 sweet potato weighing 200g/7oz
- 1 tsp olive oil
- 1 garlic clove, crushed
- ½ onion, sliced
- 2 tsp medium curry powder
- 200g/7oz tinned chopped tomatoes
- 250ml/1 cup chicken or vegetable stock
- Salt & pepper to taste

Method

1 Peel the sweet potato and use the chipper blade to turn into thick spirals.

2 Gently heat a non-stick saucepan on the hob with the olive oil and sauté the garlic & onion for a few minutes until softened.

3 Stir through the curry powder and add the chopped tomatoes & stock.

4 Gently simmer for 5 minutes or until the sweet potatoes are tender.

5 Serve and serve.

CHEFS NOTE
Chopped fresh chives makes a great garnish to this thick soup.

CHICKEN & CARROT SOUP

240 calories per serving

Ingredients

- 1 carrot weighing 200g/7oz
- 1 tsp olive oil
- 75g/3oz chicken breast, thinly sliced
- 1 stalk celery, chopped
- ½ onion, sliced
- 1 garlic clove, crushed
- ½ tsp dried thyme
- 370ml/1½ cups chicken stock
- Salt & pepper to taste

Method

1 Peel, top & tail the carrot and use the shredder blade to turn into thin noodles.

2 Gently heat a non-stick saucepan on the hob with the olive oil and sauté the sliced chicken, celery, onion & garlic for 2 minutes.

3 Add the thyme, stock and carrot noodles and simmer for approx. 3 minutes or until the noodles are tender and the chicken is cooked through.

4 Season and serve.

CHEFS NOTE

The carrots can be served raw if you prefer - just add to the soup after cooking.

COCONUT MILK NOODLE SOUP

210
calories per serving

Ingredients

- Courgettes/Zucchini weighing 300g/11oz
- 1 tsp olive oil
- ½ onion, sliced
- 1 garlic clove, crushed

- 1 tbsp green Thai curry paste
- 250ml/1 cup chicken or vegetable stock
- 120ml/½ cup low fat coconut milk
- Salt & pepper to taste

Method

1 Top & tail the courgettes and use the shredder blade to turn into thin noodles.

2 Gently heat a non-stick saucepan on the hob with the olive oil and sauté the onion & garlic for 2 minutes.

3 Stir through the curry paste. Add the stock and noodles and simmer for 2 minutes. Stir though the coconut milk and simmer for a further 2 minutes or until the soup is piping hot and noodles are tender.

4 Season and serve.

CHEFS NOTE
Try serving with a twist of lime.

CHOPPED SPIRAL VEG SOUP

290 calories per serving

Ingredients

- 1 large carrot weighing 200g/7oz
- 1 courgette/zucchini weighing 200g/7oz
- 1 tsp olive oil
- 1 stalk celery, chopped
- ½ onion, sliced
- 1 garlic clove, crushed

- ½ tsp dried basil
- 125g/5oz potato, peeled & chopped
- 370ml/1½ cups vegetable or chicken stock
- Salt & pepper to taste

Method

1 Top & tail the courgette, peel the carrot and use the shredder blade to turn into thin spirals.

2 Take a knife and, holding the spirals in bunches, roughly chop into 1cm/½ inch pieces.

3 Gently heat a non-stick saucepan on the hob with the olive oil and sauté the sliced celery, onion, garlic, basil & potatoes for a few minutes until softened. Add the stock and cook for 5 minutes.

4 Place in a blender for a few seconds and blend until smooth.

5 Return to the pan along with the chopped spiral veggies and simmer for 3-4 minutes or until the veg is tender and the soup is piping hot.

6 Season and serve.

CHEFS NOTE
Chop the spirals as roughly as you like, 1cm pieces is just a suggestion.

SHRIMP & FRESH PEA NOODLES

260 calories per serving

Ingredients

- Courgettes/Zucchini weighing 300g/11oz
- ½ onion, sliced
- ½ red pepper, deseeded & sliced
- 1 garlic clove, crushed
- A pinch of crushed dried chillies
- 150g/5oz raw, shelled king prawns/jumbo shrimp
- 1 tbsp soy sauce
- 2 tsp Thai fish sauce
- 1 tsp lime juice
- 75g/3oz fresh peas
- Low cal cooking oil spray
- Salt & pepper to taste

Method

1 Top & tail the courgettes and use the shredder blade to turn into spaghetti noodles.

2 Gently heat a large non-stick frying pan on the hob with a little low cal oil. Sauté the onion, peppers & garlic for a few minutes until softened.

3 Add the chillies, prawns, soy sauce, fish sauce & lime juice and cook for 3 minutes.

4 Add the noodles & fresh peas and move around the pan for 3-5 minutes or until everything is piping hot.

5 Season and serve.

CHEFS NOTE

Use chicken instead of prawns if you prefer.

SWEET CHILLI PRAWN 'NOODLES'

260 calories per serving

Ingredients

- Courgettes/Zucchini weighing 300g/11oz
- 1 garlic clove, crushed
- 200g/7oz raw, shelled king prawns/ jumbo shrimp
- 1 tbsp sweet chilli sauce
- 1 tsp soy sauce
- 50g/2oz spinach leaves
- Low cal cooking oil spray
- Salt & pepper to taste

Method

1 Top & tail the courgettes and use the shredder blade to turn into thin noodles.

2 Gently heat a large non-stick frying pan on the hob with a little low cal spray and sauté the garlic & prawns in the saucepan for a few minutes.

3 Add the sweet chilli sauce & soy sauce and stir well.

4 Add the courgette noodles & spinach and stir-fry for 3-4 minutes or until the prawns are cooked through and the noodles are tender

5 Season and serve.

CHEFS NOTE
Keep extra soy sauce to hand to suit your own taste.

RAW CITRUS SALAD

240
calories per serving

Ingredients

- 1 courgette/zucchini weighing 200g/7oz
- 1 sweet potato weighing 200g/7oz
- 1 tbsp lime juice
- 1 tbsp honey
- 1 tbsp olive oil
- Pinch of sea salt
- 4 spring onions/scallion, thinly sliced lengthways
- Freshly ground black pepper

Method

1 Top & tail the courgette, peel the sweet potato and use the chipper blade to turn both into thick spirals.

2 In a bowl mix together the lime juice, honey, olive oil & salt. Add the courgette & sweet potato spirals and toss together.

3 Sprinkle with the sliced spring onions and serve.

CHEFS NOTE
Crunchy, fresh & simple. Serve as a lunchtime snack or as a side to sliced grilled chicken.

SWEET ROASTED CHERRY TOMATO & ZUCCHINI SPIRALS

270 calories per serving

Ingredients

- Courgettes/Zucchini weighing 300g/11oz
- 200g/7oz ripe cherry tomatoes
- 1 tsp brown sugar (or honey)
- 2 garlic cloves, crushed

- ½ onion, chopped
- 1 tbsp olive oil
- 1 tbsp freshly chopped basil
- Low cal cooking oil spray
- Salt & pepper to taste

Method

1 Preheat the oven to 200c/400f/Gas 6.

2 Halve the cherry tomatoes, place on a baking tray, spray with a little low cal oil and sprinkle with sugar. Put into the oven and cook for about 20 minutes or until they are roasted and soft.

3 Meanwhile top & tail the courgettes and use the chipper blade to turn into thick spirals.

4 Gently heat a large non-stick frying pan on the hob with the garlic, onion & olive oil and sauté for a few minutes until softened.

5 Add the spirals and move around the pan for 3-5 minutes or until everything is piping hot. Toss through the sweet roasted tomatoes and pile into a shallow bowl.

6 Sprinkle with basil. Season and serve.

CHEFS NOTE
Vine ripened plum tomatoes will work just as well but you may need to roast for a little longer.

SERVES 1

CAJUN SWEET POTATO CURLS

290 calories per serving

Ingredients

- **1 sweet potato weighing 200g/7oz**
- **1 tbsp olive oil**
- **½ tsp each sea salt, cumin, paprika & garlic powder**
- **Salt & pepper to taste**

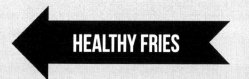

HEALTHY FRIES

Method

1 Preheat the oven to 200c/400f/Gas 6.

2 Use the chipper blade to turn into thick potato curls, don't bother peeling the sweet potato.

3 Place everything in a bowl and combine really well to ensure every curl is coated with seasoning and oil.

4 Arrange on a non-stick baking tray and spread out to make one layer. Place in the oven and cook for about 20 minutes, turning once.

5 Season and serve.

CHEFS NOTE

Keep an eye on the curls when they are cooking as they can burn easily. Reduce the heat if you find this happening.

CUMIN CARROT & CITRUS SALAD

295 calories per serving

Ingredients

- Carrots weighing 300g/11oz
- 1 orange
- 1 tbsp orange juice
- 1 tbsp olive oil
- 2 tsp lemon juice
- 1 tbsp olive oil

- ½ tsp ground cumin
- ½ tsp brown sugar
- Pinch of sea salt
- 50g/2oz baby spinach leaves
- 1 tbsp freshly chopped coriander/cilantro
- Freshly ground black pepper

Method

1 Top, tail & peel the carrots and use the shredder blade to turn into thin spirals.

2 Peel the orange, divide into segments and chop into chunks.

3 In a bowl toss mix together the orange juice, oil, lemon juice, cumin, sugar & salt to make a dressing.

4 Toss the carrot spirals and orange pieces in the dressing.

5 Place the spinach in a shallow bowl and arrange carrot & orange on top. Sprinkle over the coriander, season and serve.

CHEFS NOTE
This salad is also good with fresh mint instead of coriander.

SWEET POTATO & SWEET PEPPER SAUCE

260 calories per serving

Ingredients

- 1 sweet potato weighing 200g/7oz
- 1 garlic clove
- 1-2 tbsp water
- 1 tbsp tomato puree/paste
- 3 roasted peppers, from a jar
- ½ tsp dried basil
- Low cal cooking oil spray
- Salt & pepper to taste

Method

1 Peel the sweet potato and use the chipper blade to turn into thick spirals.

2 Cook the spirals in salted boiling water for 2-3 minutes. Drain and put to one side.

3 Place the garlic, water, puree, peppers & basil into a mini blender and blend until smooth (or finely chop everything together and combine if you don't have a mini blender).

4 Gently heat a large non-stick frying pan on the hob with a little low cal spray, add the pepper sauce and cook for a couple of minutes. Add the spirals to the pan, combine well and cook until everything is piping hot

5 Check the seasoning and serve.

CHEFS NOTE
Fresh chopped basil complements this dish perfectly.

CILANTRO SWEET POTATO SPIRALS

210 calories per serving

Ingredients

- 1 sweet potato weighing 200g/7oz
- ½ red onion, sliced
- ½ tsp ground coriander/cilantro
- Large pinch of sea salt
- 2 tbsp freshly chopped coriander/cilantro
- Low cal cooking oil spray
- Salt & pepper to taste

Method

1 Peel the sweet potato and use the chipper blade to turn into thick spirals.

2 Cook the spirals in salted boiling water for 2-3 minutes. Drain and put to one side.

3 Gently heat a large non-stick frying pan on the hob with a little low cal spray, add the onions and cook for a few minutes until softened.

4 Stir through the ground coriander & salt and cook for a minute longer (add a splash of water if you need to loosen the pan up).

5 Add the spirals to the pan with a little more low cal spray, combine well and cook for a few minutes until everything is piping hot.

6 Stir through the chopped coriander. Check the seasoning and serve.

CHEFS NOTE
This is a quick and easy lunch for one or side dish for two.

FETA CHEESE 'SPAGHETTI'

240 calories per serving

Ingredients

- Courgettes/Zucchini weighing 300g/11oz
- 1 tsp olive oil
- 1 garlic clove, crushed
- 1 tbsp pine nuts
- 4 spring onions/scallions, finely sliced
- 50g/2oz low fat Feta cheese, crumbled
- Salt & pepper to taste

Method

1 Top & tail the courgettes and use the shredder blade to turn into spaghetti noodles.

2 Gently heat a large non-stick frying pan on the hob with the olive oil and sauté the garlic for a minute or two until softened.

3 Add the spaghetti noodles & pine nuts and move around the pan for 3-5 minutes or until everything is piping hot.

4 Tip the 'pasta' into a bowl. Sprinkle over crumbled the feta cheese and spring onions.

5 Season and serve.

CHEFS NOTE
Try serving with a little freshly chopped mint.

PESTO YOGURT EGG PLANT

225
calories per
serving

Ingredients

- 1 aubergine/egg plant weighing 300g/11oz
- ½ red onion, sliced
- 1 tsp olive oil
- 1 garlic clove, crushed
- Pinch of crushed chillies
- 1 tbsp fat free Greek yogurt
- 2 tsp green pesto
- 1 baby gem/cos lettuce shredded
- Salt & pepper to taste

Method

1 Top & tail the aubergine and use the slicer blade to turn into ribbons.

2 Gently heat the oil in a large non-stick frying pan on the hob.

3 Add the onion, garlic, aubergine ribbons & crushed chillies to the pan. Combine well and cook for 4-6 minutes or until the aubergines are cooked though.

4 Meanwhile mix together the yogurt and pesto to make a dressing.

5 Tip the aubergines and onions onto the shredded lettuce.

6 Dollop the pesto yogurt on top and serve.

CHEFS NOTE
Use more or less crushed chillies to suit your own taste.

TUNA & CHILLI 'PASTA'

220 calories per serving

Ingredients

- Courgettes/Zucchini weighing 300g/11oz
- 1 tsp olive oil
- ½ garlic clove, crushed
- ½ red chilli, deseeded & finely chopped
- ½ red onion, sliced
- 75g/3oz tinned tuna, drained
- 120ml/½ cup tomato pasatta/sauce
- Salt & pepper to taste

Method

1 Top & tail the courgettes and use the shredder blade to turn into spaghetti noodles.

2 Gently heat a large non-stick frying pan on the hob with the olive oil and sauté the garlic, chilli & onion for a few minutes until softened (add a splash of water to the pan if it needs loosening up).

3 Meanwhile gently warm the pasatta in a small pan with the tinned tuna and a pinch of salt for a few minutes.

4 Add the spaghetti noodles to the onion pan and move for 3-5 minutes or until everything is piping hot.

5 Tip the noodles into a bowl, pour over the tuna sauce. Season and serve.

CHEFS NOTE
Fresh tuna would be great too!

SAUTÉED SWEET POTATOES WITH YOGURT DRESSING

250 calories per serving

Ingredients

- 1 sweet potato weighing 200g/7oz
- ½ red onion, sliced
- 1 garlic clove, crushed
- ½ tsp paprika
- 2 tsp honey
- 1 tsp balsamic vinegar
- Large pinch of sea salt
- 1 tbsp fat free Greek yoghurt
- Low cal cooking oil spray
- Salt & pepper to taste

Method

1 Peel the sweet potato and use the chipper blade to turn into thick spirals.

2 Cook the spirals in salted boiling water for 2-3 minutes. Drain and put to one side.

3 Gently heat a large non-stick frying pan on the hob with a little low cal spray. Add the onions & garlic and cook for a few minutes until softened.

4 Stir through the paprika, balsamic vinegar and 1 teaspoon of the honey.

5 Cook for a minute longer before adding the spirals to the pan. Combine well and cook for 3-4 minutes on a medium high heat until everything turns golden brown and is piping hot (add a splash of water if you need to loosen the pan up).

6 Tip the spirals into a shallow bowl. Mix together the remaining teaspoon of honey with the yogurt and drizzle over the top of the spirals.

CHEFS NOTE
Try some chopped mint in the yogurt dressing too.

SIMPLE MINT & OLIVE ZUCHINNI SALAD

210 calories per serving

Ingredients

- Courgettes/Zucchini weighing 300g/11oz
- 6 pitted black olives, finely chopped
- 6 cherry tomatoes, finely chopped
- Zest & juice of ¼ lemon
- 1 tbsp olive oil
- Pinch of salt
- 1 tbsp freshly chopped mint
- Salt & pepper to taste

Method

1 Top & tail the courgettes and use the slicer/ straight blade to turn into ribbons.

2 In a bowl mix together the olives, chopped tomatoes, zest, lemon juice, olive oil, salt and mint to make a dressing.

3 Add the ribbons to the bowl and toss together so that everything is thoroughly coated with the dressing.

4 Season and serve.

CHEFS NOTE
This is even better chilled and left to marinade for 20 minutes.

SPICED SPINACH & SPIRALIZED SWEET POTATOES

240 calories per serving

Ingredients

- 1 sweet potato weighing 200g/7oz
- ½ onion, sliced
- ½ tsp freshly grated ginger
- 1 garlic clove, crushed
- 1 tsp garam masala
- ½ red chilli, deseeded & finely sliced
- 100g/3½oz spinach
- 1 tbsp low fat/half and half cream
- Low cal cooking oil spray
- Salt & pepper to taste

Method

1 Peel the sweet potato and use the chipper blade to turn into thick spirals.

2 Cook the spirals in salted boiling water for 2-3 minutes. Drain and put to one side.

3 Gently heat a large non-stick frying pan on the hob with a little low cal spray. Add the onions, ginger, garlic, garam masala & chopped chilli and cook for a few minutes until softened (add a splash of water to the pan if you need to loosen it up).

4 Add the sweet potato spirals and spinach to the pan and cook until the potatoes are piping hot and the spinach is wilted.

5 Remove from the heat, stir through the cream and serve immediately.

CHEFS NOTE
Use curry powder if you don't have garam masala.

ANCHOVY & CHILLI 'PASTA'

220 calories per serving

Ingredients

- Courgettes/Zucchini weighing 300g/11oz
- 2 tsp olive oil
- 5 anchovy fillets, drained
- ½ onion, sliced
- ½ tsp crushed chilli flakes
- 2 tsp lemon juice
- ½ tsp dried thyme
- Salt & pepper to taste

Method

1 Top & tail the courgettes and use the shredder blade to turn into spaghetti noodles.

2 Gently heat a large non-stick frying pan on the hob with the olive oil.

3 Add the anchovy fillets and onions and sauté for a few minutes until softened.

4 Add the chilli flakes, lemon juice & thyme and continue cooking & stirring until the anchovy fillets begin to dissolve.

5 Add the spaghetti noodles and move around the pan for 3-5 minutes or until everything is piping hot.

6 Season and serve.

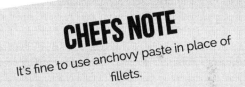

CHEFS NOTE
It's fine to use anchovy paste in place of fillets.

CARROT & PARMA SALAD

290 calories per serving

Ingredients

- Carrots weighing 300g/11oz
- 1 tbsp freshly chopped flat leaf parsley
- 1 tbsp olive oil
- 2 spring onions/scallions, sliced lengthways

- 2 slices Parma ham
- 50g/2oz rocket leaves
- Pinch of sea salt
- Freshly ground black pepper

Method

1 Top, tail & peel the carrots and use the shredder blade to turn into thin spirals.

2 In a bowl toss together the spirals, chopped parsley, olive oil, spring onions & sea salt.

3 Arrange the rocket leaves on a plate. Place the ham over the leaves and tip the carrot salad on top.

4 Season with lots of black pepper and serve.

CHEFS NOTE
Try serving the salad with a twist of lemon juice.

THE *Skinny*
SPIRALIZER

UNDER 400 CALORIES

BEEF KEEMA

360
calories per serving

Ingredients

- 1 courgette/zucchini weighing 200g/11oz
- 1 carrot weighing 200g/11oz
- 1 tsp olive oil
- ½ onion, sliced
- 1 garlic clove, crushed
- 125g/4oz lean mince/ground beef

- ½ tsp garam masala
- 1 tsp turmeric
- Large pinch of sea salt
- 100g/3½oz tinned chopped tomatoes
- Low cal cooking oil spray
- Salt & pepper to taste

Method

1 Peel the carrot. Top & tail the courgette & carrot and use the shredder blade to turn both into thin spirals.

2 Heat a non-stick frying pan with the olive oil and sauté the onion & garlic for a few minutes. Add the beef and brown for a couple of minutes.

3 Stir through the garam masala, turmeric & salt and cook for 2 minutes. Add the tomatoes and spirals.

4 Cover and leave to simmer for 5 minutes or until the beef is cooked through and the spirals are tender. Season and serve.

CHEFS NOTE
Chopped coriander and chillies make a good garnish for this simple Indian dish.

SWEET GROUND BEEF & ZUCCHINI TWIRLS

390 calories per serving

Ingredients

- 1 large courgette/zuchinni weighing 300g/11oz
- 1 tbsp olive oil
- ½ red chilli, deseeded & finely chopped
- Zest & juice of ½ lime
- Large pinch of sea salt
- ½ onion, sliced

- 1 garlic clove, crushed
- ½ red pepper, deseeded & sliced
- 125g/4oz lean ground/mince beef
- 1 tsp honey
- 1 tbsp tomato ketchup
- Low cal cooking oil spray
- Salt & pepper to taste

Method

1 Top & tail the courgette and use the slicer/straight blade to turn into ribbons.

2 Place the ribbons in a bowl with the olive oil, chilli, lime juice, zest, and salt. Combine really well to coat every inch of the courgette in the olive oil and leave to marinade while you cook the beef.

3 Heat a non-stick frying pan with a little low cal oil. Sauté the onion, garlic & sliced peppers for a few minutes until softened.

4 Add the beef and brown for 2 minutes.

5 Stir through the honey and ketchup and continue cooking for 4-5 minutes or until the beef is cooked through .

6 Place the zesty ribbons on top and serve.

CHEFS NOTE
Use very lean, ideally organic, beef.

CHICKEN & COURGETTE SKEWERS

360 calories per serving

Ingredients

- Courgettes/Zucchini weighing 300g/11oz
- 1 tbsp olive oil
- ½ red chilli, deseeded & finely chopped
- Zest & juice of ½ lime
- Large pinch of sea salt
- 125g/4oz chicken breast, cubed
- 1 tsp honey
- Low cal cooking oil spray
- Metal kebab skewers
- Salt & pepper to taste

Method

1 Preheat the grill to a medium/high heat.

2 Top & Tail the courgettes and use the slicer/ straight blade to turn into ribbons.

3 Place the ribbons in a bowl with the olive oil, chilli, lime juice, zest, and salt. Combine really well to coat every inch of the courgette in the olive oil.

4 Meanwhile season the chicken and, in a bowl, combine with the honey.

5 Place the chicken cubes and courgettes in turn on the skewers to make 1 large or two smaller kebabs.

6 Place under the preheated grill and, turning occasionally, cook for 8-10 minutes or until the chicken is cooked through.

CHEFS NOTE
Skewer the ribbons by weaving them concertina style on the kebab sticks.

CREAMY THAI VEG NOODLES

320 calories per serving

Ingredients

- 1 courgette/zucchini weighing 150g/5oz
- 1 carrot weighing 150g/5oz
- 1 garlic clove, crushed
- 1 tsp grated ginger
- 1 tsp lemon juice
- 1 tbsp soy sauce
- ½ ripe avocado
- 60ml/¼ cup water
- Low cal cooking oil spray
- Salt & pepper to taste

Method

1 Top & tail the courgette. Peel the carrot and use the shredder blade to turn both into thin noodles.

2 Gently heat a large non-stick frying pan on the hob with a little low cal oil.

3 Add the courgette noodles and move around the pan for 3-5 minutes or until tender (add a splash of water to the pan if you need to).

4 Meanwhile place all the other ingredients, except the carrot, into a mini blender to make a creamy dressing (or mash everything together with a fork if you don't have one).

5 Take the pan off the heat. Stir through the creamy dressing and toss the carrot through.

6 Season and serve.

CHEFS NOTE
The raw carrots give this dish a nice crunch, it's fine to sauté though if you prefer.

PRAWN & CHILLI STIR-FRY

300
calories per serving

Ingredients

- Carrots weighing 300g/11oz
- 2 tsp olive oil
- 1 garlic clove, crushed
- ½ red chilli, deseeded & finely chopped
- ½ onion, chopped

- 75g/3oz trimmed green beans
- 150g/5oz raw, shelled king prawns/ jumbo shrimp
- Salt & pepper to taste

Method

1 Top, tail & peel the carrots and use the straight/ slicer blade to turn into thin ribbons.

2 Gently heat a large non-stick frying pan on the hob with the olive oil and sauté the garlic, chilli & onions for 2 minutes.

3 Add the prawns & green beans and cook for two minutes longer.

4 Add the carrot ribbons and quickly move around the pan for 2 minutes or until the prawns are cooked through.

5 Season and serve.

CHEFS NOTE
This is great served with a garnish of fresh oregano.

FRESH TUNA STIR-FRY

360 calories per serving

Ingredients

- Carrots weighing 300g/11oz
- 75g/3oz asparagus spears
- 150g/5oz fresh tuna steak
- 1 tbsp soy sauce
- 1 tsp honey

- 1 tsp lime juice
- 2 radishes, sliced
- 1 handful watercress
- Salt & pepper to taste

Method

1 Top, tail & peel the carrots and use the straight/ slicer blade to turn into thin ribbons.

2 Gently heat a large non-stick frying pan on the hob with the olive oil and sauté the carrots and asparagus for 2 minutes.

3 Make some room in the pan, add the tuna steak and cook for 1 minute each side (pile the veg on top of the tuna steak if you find it's cooking too fast)

4 Meanwhile mix together the soy sauce, honey & lime juice and pour this over the tuna and veg.

5 Tip everything onto a plate with the watercress on the side. Season and serve.

CHEFS NOTE
Increase the cooking time for the tuna if you don't want rare steak.

VEGGIE LIME & CASHEW STIR-FRY

375 calories per serving

Ingredients

- Carrots weighing 300g/11oz
- Courgettes/Zucchini weighing 300g/11oz
- 2 tsp olive oil
- 1 garlic clove, crushed
- 1 tsp freshly grated ginger
- ½ onion, chopped
- ½ red pepper, deseeded & sliced
- 125g/2oz mangetout/sugar snap peas
- 1 tsp honey
- 1 tbsp soy sauce
- 3 spring onions/scallions, chopped
- 1 tbsp fresh cashew nuts, chopped
- Lime wedges to serve
- Salt & pepper to taste

Method

1 Top & tail the carrots & courgettes. Peel the carrots and use the shredder blade to turn both into thin spiral threads.

2 Gently heat a large non-stick frying pan on the hob with the olive oil and sauté the garlic, ginger, onion, peppers & mangetout for 5 minutes until softened (add a splash of water to the pan if you need to loosen it up).

3 Stir through the honey & soy sauce and increase the heat.

4 Add the carrots & courgettes and move around the pan for approx. 4 minutes or until tender.

5 Tip everything into a shallow bowl, sprinkle over the chopped spring onions and cashew nuts. Season and serve with lime wedges.

CHEFS NOTE
Try toasting whole cashew nuts in a dry pan on a gentle heat for a minute or two until golden brown.

DRESSED CARROT & PARMESAN SALAD

360 calories per serving

Ingredients

- Carrots weighing 300g/11oz
- 1 tbsp horseradish sauce
- 1 tsp Dijon mustard
- 1 tbsp olive oil
- 1 tbsp balsamic vinegar
- Pinch of sea salt
- 50g/2oz spinach
- 25g/1oz Parmesan cheese shavings
- Freshly ground black pepper

Method

1 Top, tail & peel the carrots and use the shredder blade to turn into thin spirals.

2 In a bowl mix together the horseradish sauce, mustard, oil, vinegar & salt. Add the carrot spirals and toss together.

3 Place the spinach leaves in a shallow bowl Load the dressed salad on top and arrange the Parmesan shavings.

CHEFS NOTE
Use less horseradish if you want to reduce the heat!

CARROT, APPLE & CHEDDAR SALAD

320 calories per serving

Ingredients

- Carrots weighing 300g/11oz
- 1 eating apple
- 1 tbsp olive oil
- 1 tsp cider vinegar
- Pinch of sea salt
- 1 tbsp freshly chopped chives
- 3 spring onions/scallions, chopped
- 25g/1oz low fat grated cheddar cheese
- Freshly ground black pepper

Method

1 Top, tail & peel the carrots and use the shredder blade to turn into thin spirals.

2 Peel & core the apple and use the straight/slicer blade to turn into thin slices/ribbons.

3 In a bowl toss together the carrots, apple, oil, vinegar & salt until everything is well combined.

4 Place in a shallow bowl and sprinkle over the chives, spring onions & grated cheese.

5 Season with lots of black pepper and serve.

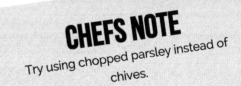

CHEFS NOTE
Try using chopped parsley instead of chives.

CHUNKY CHICKPEA 'PASTA'

310 calories per serving

Ingredients

- Courgettes/Zucchini weighing 300g/11oz
- ½ onion, chopped
- 1 garlic clove, crushed
- 200g/7oz tinned chickpeas, drained
- 250ml/1 cup vegetable stock
- Low cal cooking oil spray
- Salt & pepper to taste

Method

1 Top & tail the courgettes and use the shredder blade to turn into spaghetti noodles.

2 Heat a large non-stick frying pan on the hob with a little low cal spray and gently sauté the onions & garlic for a few minutes until softened.

3 Meanwhile gently warm the chickpeas in a small pan with the stock.

4 Tip the sautéed onions into a blender and use a slotted spoon to add the chickpeas too. Add about half the stock and pulse for a second at a time until you have a chunky sauce. Add more of the stock to alter the consistency if you want.

5 Add the spaghetti noodles to the empty frying pan and move around the pan for 3-5 minutes or until they are piping hot. Tip over the chickpea sauce.

6 Combine well. Season and serve.

CHEFS NOTE
Garnish with chopped flat leaf parsley.

BEAN & HALLOUMI RIBBON SALAD

397 calories per serving

Ingredients

- Courgettes/Zucchini weighing 300g/11oz
- 125g/4oz tinned Borlotti beans, rinsed & drained
- Zest & juice of ¼ lemon
- 1 tbsp olive oil
- Pinch of salt
- 50g/2oz sliced low fat halloumi cheese
- 1 tbsp freshly chopped coriander/cilantro
- Salt & pepper to taste

Method

1 Preheat the grill to a medium/high heat

2 Top & tail the courgettes and use the slicer/straight blade to turn into ribbons.

3 Toss the ribbons in a bowl with the borlotti beans, zest, lemon juice, olive oil & salt.

4 Place the halloumi slices under the grill and cook for a minute or two on each side until bubbling and golden brown.

5 Tip the courgette and bean salad into a bowl. Place the grilled cheese on top and sprinkle with chopped coriander.

6 Season and serve.

CHEFS NOTE
Borlotti beans are good but use any type of tinned bean you prefer.

SWEET POTATO & PORCINI SPIRALS

380 calories per serving

Ingredients

- 1 sweet potato weighing 200g/7oz
- 25g/1oz dried porcini mushrooms
- 2 tsp low fat 'butter' spread
- 1 tbsp plain/all purpose flour
- 250ml/1 cup semi skimmed/half fat milk
- ½ tsp dried thyme
- Low cal cooking oil spray
- Salt & pepper to taste

Method

1 Peel the sweet potato and use the chipper blade to turn into thick spirals.

2 Place the porcini mushrooms in a little warm water to rehydrate for a few minutes while you cook the spirals in salted boiling water for 2-3 minutes. Drain the spirals and put to one side.

3 Gently heat the 'butter' in a saucepan and, when it's melted, add the flour. Mix this together to form a roux (paste).

4 Whilst still on the heat take a whisk and gently add the milk and thyme whisking the roux all the time to make sure you end with a smooth sauce.

5 When the sauce thickens up remove from the heat.

6 Meanwhile drain and finely chop the rehydrated mushrooms.

7 Gently heat a large non-stick frying pan on the hob with a little low cal spray and add the mushrooms, spirals & sauce to the frying pan.

8 Combine well and cook for a few minutes until everything is piping hot

9 Check the seasoning and serve.

CHEFS NOTE

Adjust the chilli to suit your own taste..

SKINNY SAUSAGE & SPINACH 'SPAGHETTI'

375 calories per serving

Ingredients

- Courgettes/Zucchini weighing 300g/11oz
- 150g/5oz venison sausage
- 1 garlic clove, crushed
- ½ onion, sliced
- 250ml/1 cup tomato passata/sauce
- 1 tbsp tomato puree/paste
- ½ tsp each salt & brown sugar
- 1 tsp Worcestershire sauce/A1 steak sauce
- 75g/3oz spinach
- Low cal cooking oil spray
- Salt & pepper to taste

Method

1 Top & tail the courgettes and use the shredder blade to turn into spaghetti noodles.

2 Gently heat a large non-stick frying pan on the hob with a little low cal spray.

3 Add the sausages, garlic & onions to the pan and cook for about 8-10 minutes or until the sausages are cooked through (add a splash of water to the pan if you need to loosen it up).

4 Meanwhile combine the passata/sauce, puree, salt, sugar and Worcestershire/A1 sauce in a pan and gently cook on a low heat.

5 When they're ready slice the sausages into discs and add these, along with the onions, to the passata/sauce pan.

6 Use the empty frying pan to gently saulé the spaghetti noodles and spinach. Move about the pan for a couple of minutes until piping hot.

7 Tip the noodles and spinach into a bowl. Pour over the sausages & sauce.

8 Season and serve.

CHEFS NOTE
Chicken or turkey sausages are also a good skinny sausage alternative.

PESTO CHICKEN 'PASTA'

320 calories per serving

Ingredients

- Courgettes/Zucchini weighing 300g/11oz
- ½ onion, sliced
- 100g/3½oz chicken breast, sliced
- 1 tbsp green pesto sauce
- 2 tsp grated Parmesan cheese
- Low cal cooking oil spray
- Salt & pepper to taste

Method

1 Top & tail the courgettes and use the shredder blade to turn into spaghetti noodles.

2 Gently heat a large non-stick frying pan on the hob with a little low cal spray.

3 Add the onions and sliced chicken and cook for a few minutes until the onions are softened and the chicken is cooked through.

4 Stir through the pesto and then add the spaghetti noodles. Move about the pan for a couple of minutes until everything is well combined and piping hot (add a splash of water to the pan if you need to loosen it up).

5 Tip into a bowl, sprinkle over the Parmesan cheese, season and serve.

CHEFS NOTE

Jars of reduced fat pesto are now available which will help shave off a few extra calories.

SWEET POTATO CARBONARA

320
calories per serving

Ingredients

- 1 sweet potato weighing 200g/7oz
- 1 slice lean, back bacon/Canadian bacon
- 50g/2oz fresh peas
- 60ml/ ¼ cup low fat cream
- ½ free range egg
- 1 tsp grated Parmesan cheese
- Low cal cooking oil spray
- Salt & pepper to taste

Method

1 Peel the sweet potato and use the shredder blade to turn into spiralized potato noodles.

2 Cook the noodles in salted boiling water for 1-1 ½ minutes. Drain and put to one side.

3 Gently heat a large non-stick frying pan on the hob with a little low cal spray and cook the bacon for a couple of minutes. When it's ready remove from the pan and finely slice.

4 Add the noodles, peas & chopped bacon and move about the pan for 3-4 minutes or until everything is piping hot (add a splash of water to the pan if you need to loosen it up).

5 In a cup gently beat together the cream, egg and Parmesan cheese. Pour this into the pan and combine everything over a gentle heat (this only needs 30 sec-1 min, you don't want scrambled egg).

6 Tip into a bowl, season with black pepper and serve.

CHEFS NOTE
Frozen peas are fine to use too. Just cook for a minute or two in boiling water before adding to the pan with the potato noodles.

THE *Skinny*
SPIRALIZER

UNDER 500 CALORIES

GRILLED CHICKEN & DOLCELATTE SPIRALS

420 calories per serving

Ingredients

- 125g/4oz chicken breast
- Courgettes/Zucchini weighing 300g/11oz
- 2 tsp olive oil
- 4 cherry tomatoes, halved
- 1 garlic clove, crushed
- 25g/1oz dolcelatte cheese
- Low cal cooking oil spray
- Salt & pepper to taste

Method

1 Preheat the grill.

2 Season the chicken, spray with a little low cal oil and cook under the grill for 10-12 minutes or until cooked through.

3 Meanwhile top & tail the courgettes and use the shredder blade to turn into thin spirals.

4 Gently heat a large non-stick frying pan on the hob with the olive oil and sauté the garlic & tomatoes for a few minutes until softened.

5 Add the courgette noodles and stir-fry for 4-5 minutes. Arrange on a plate and crumble over the dolcelatte cheese.

7 Cut the grilled chicken into thick slices and place on top.

8 Season and serve.

CHEFS NOTE
Feta cheese makes a good alternative to dolcelatte.

6

CHICKEN & PEPPER 'NOODLE' STIR-FRY

420 calories per serving

Ingredients

- Courgettes/Zucchini weighing 300g/11oz
- 2 tsp olive oil
- 150g/5oz chicken breast, thinly sliced
- 1 garlic clove, crushed
- ½ onion, chopped
- 1 red pepper, deseeded & sliced
- 60ml/½ cup chicken stock
- 1 tbsp soy sauce
- Salt & pepper to taste

Method

1 Top & tail the courgettes and use the shredder blade to turn into noodles.

2 Gently heat a large non-stick frying pan on the hob with the olive oil and sauté the sliced chicken, garlic, onion & peppers for 3 minutes until softened.

3 Add the stock & soy sauce, increase the heat and cook for 2-3 minutes to reduce about half of the stock.

4 Add the noodles and move around the pan for 3-5 minutes or until the courgette noodles are tender and the chicken is cooked through.

5 Season and serve.

CHEFS NOTE
Add extra veg if you like: tenderstem broccoli/broccolini and sugar snap peas make good additions.

HONEY CHICKEN & CRUNCHY CARROT STIR-FRY

460 calories per serving

Ingredients

- Carrots weighing 300g/11oz
- 2 tsp olive oil
- 150g/5oz chicken breast, thinly sliced
- 1 garlic clove, crushed
- 1 tsp freshly grated ginger
- ½ onion, chopped

- 125g/2oz tenderstem broccoli/ broccolini, finely chopped
- 1 tsp clear honey
- 1 tsp lime juice
- 1 tbsp soy sauce
- Salt & pepper to taste

Method

1 Peel, top & tail the carrots and use the shredder blade to turn into thin threads.

2 Gently heat a large non-stick frying pan on the hob with the olive oil and sauté the chicken, garlic, ginger, onion & broccoli for 5 minutes until softened (add a splash of water to the pan if you need to loosen it up).

3 Stir through the honey, lime juice & soy sauce and increase the heat. Add the carrots and move around the pan for 2 minutes or until the chicken is cooked through.

4 Season and serve.

CHEFS NOTE
The carrots will have a little crunch left but you could have them raw piled on top if you prefer.

SWEET POTATO WITH SPANISH SAUCE

405
calories per serving

Ingredients

- 1 sweet potato weighing 200g/7oz
- ¼ red onion, sliced
- 1 garlic clove, crushed
- 50g/2oz sliced chorizo sausage, chopped
- 2 tbsp tomato puree/paste
- ½ tsp paprika
- 120ml/½ cup red wine
- Low cal cooking oil spray
- Salt & pepper to taste

Method

1 Peel the sweet potato and use the chipper blade to turn into thick spirals.

2 Cook the spirals in salted boiling water for 2-3 minutes. Drain and put to one side.

3 Meanwhile gently heat a large non-stick frying pan on the hob with a little low cal spray. Add the onions, garlic & chorizo and gently sauté for a few minutes until softened.

4 Stir through the puree and paprika. Add the wine and increase the heat until the wine begins to boil.

5 Reduce the heat and simmer for about 5 minutes or until the wine has reduced down by half.

6 Add the spirals to the frying pan. Combine well and cook for a few minutes until everything is piping hot.

7 Check the seasoning and serve.

CHEFS NOTE
Use chicken stock in place of wine if you wish.

BAKED SWEET POTATO 'MACARONI' CHEESE

450 calories per serving

Ingredients

- 1 sweet potato weighing 200g/7oz
- 2 tsp low fat 'butter' spread
- 1 tbsp plain/all purpose flour
- 250ml/1 cup semi skimmed/half fat milk
- 50g/2oz low fat grated cheese
- Pinch of ground nutmeg
- Salt & pepper to taste

Method

1 Preheat the oven to 200c/400f/Gas 6.

2 Peel the sweet potato and use the chipper blade to turn into thick spirals.

3 Cook the spirals in salted boiling water for 2-3 minutes. Drain and put to one side.

4 Gently heat the butter in a saucepan and, when it's melted, add the flour. Mix this together to form a roux (paste).

5 Whilst still on the heat take a whisk and gently add the milk whisking the roux all the time to make sure you end with a smooth sauce. When the sauce thickens up add the cheese & nutmeg and remove from the heat.

6 In an oven proof dish combine the spirals and cheese sauce. Place in the oven and cook for 20 minutes or until golden brown and cooked through.

7 Check the seasoning and serve.

CHEFS NOTE
This is lovely served with a crisp green salad.

CHICKEN & SESAME CUCUMBER NOODLES

480 calories per serving

Ingredients

- 1 cucumber
- 2 tbsp olive oil
- 1 tsp sesame oil
- 1 tsp freshly grated ginger
- 2 tbsp soy sauce
- 8 spring onions/scallions, finely chopped
- 150g/5oz cooked chicken breast, shredded
- 75g/3oz asparagus spears, thickly sliced
- Pinch of dried crushed chillies
- Salt & pepper to taste

Method

1 Top, tail & peel the cucumber and use the shredder blade to turn into thin noodles.

2 Mix together the olive oil, sesame oil, ginger and soy sauce to make a dressing.

3 Plunge the asparagus in salted boiling water and cook for two minutes. Drain and refresh in a sieve with cold water.

4 Combine the asparagus and spring onions with the dressing. Toss with the cucumber noodles and load the shredded chicken over the top.

5 Sprinkle with crushed chillies and serve.

CHEFS NOTE
Add more soy sauce and chillies if you wish.

COCONUT THAI CURRY

499 calories per serving

Ingredients

- 1 sweet potato, weighing 300g/11oz
- 1 tsp olive oil
- 1 garlic clove, crushed
- 1 tsp freshly grated ginger
- ½ onion, sliced
- ½ red pepper, deseeded & sliced
- 1 tbsp red Thai curry paste
- 60ml/¼ cup low fat coconut milk
- 125g/4oz chicken breast, thinly sliced
- Salt & pepper to taste

Method

1 Peel the sweet potato and use the shredder blade to turn into thin noodles.

2 In a non-stick frying pan heat the olive oil and gently sauté the garlic, ginger, onion & sliced peppers for a few minutes until softened.

3 Add the curry paste and chicken and cook for 3 minutes.

4 Add the sweet potato noodles, stir through the coconut milk and cook for 5 minutes or until the chicken is cooked through and the noodles are tender.

5 Season and serve.

CHEFS NOTE

Garnish with some chopped coriander or flat leaf parsley.

SHRIMP & MISO

405
calories per serving

Ingredients

- 1 cucumber
- 1 tbsp olive oil
- 2 garlic cloves, crushed
- ½ onion, sliced
- 75g/3oz sugar snap peas
- 75g/3oz tenderstem broccoli/broccolini

- 200g/7oz raw, shelled king prawns/ jumbo shrimp
- 1 tbsp soy sauce
- 2 tsp tsp miso paste
- 120ml/½ cup vegetable stock
- Salt & pepper to taste
-

Method

1 Top & tail the cucumber and use the shredder blade to turn into thin noodles.

2 Gently heat a non-stick saucepan on the hob with the olive oil and sauté the garlic, sliced onion, peas, broccoli for 4 minutes.

3 Add the prawns, soy sauce, miso paste & stock and simmer for 5 minutes or until the prawns are pink and cooked through.

4 Quickly stir through the cucumber noodles, just long enough to take the chill off them. Drain off any excess liquid from the pan and serve in a shallow bowl.

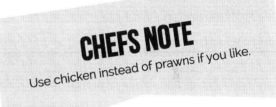

CHEFS NOTE

Use chicken instead of prawns if you like.

SWEET POTATO RAGU

485 calories per serving

Ingredients

- 1 sweet potato weighing 200g/11oz
- 1 tsp olive oil
- ½ onion, sliced
- 1 garlic clove, crushed
- 125g/4oz lean mince/ground beef
- 200g/7oz tinned chopped tomatoes
- ½ tsp dried thyme or oregano
- 1 tsp Worcestershire sauce/A1 steak sauce
- 1 tbsp tomato puree/paste
- 60ml/¼ cup vegetable stock
- Low cal cooking oil spray
- Salt & pepper to taste

Method

1 Peel the sweet potato and use the chipper blade to turn into thick spirals.

2 Heat a non-stick frying pan with the olive oil and sauté the onion & garlic for a few minutes. Add the beef and brown for a couple of minutes.

3 Stir through the chopped tomatoes, thyme, Worcestershire sauce, puree & stock.

4 Increase the heat a little and leave to simmer for 10-15 minutes, stirring coocasionally.

5 Meanwhile cook the sweet potato spirals in salted boiling water for 1-2 minutes.

6 Drain and place in a bowl with the ragu beef poured over the top.

7 Season and serve.

CHEFS NOTE
Stir the cooked sweet potatoes through the ragu before serving if you prefer it that way.

RED PESTO SPIRALS

480 calories per serving

Ingredients

- 1 sweet potato weighing 200g/7oz
- 150g/5oz cooked chicken breast, shredded
- ½ onion, chopped
- 1 garlic clove, crushed
- 1 tbsp red pesto sauce
- 2 plum tomatoes, quartered
- 2 tsp grated Parmesan cheese
- Low cal cooking oil spray
- Salt & pepper to taste

Method

1 Peel the sweet potato and use the chipper blade to turn into thick spirals.

2 Heat a non-stick frying pan with the olive oil and sauté the onion & garlic for a few minutes.

3 Meanwhile cook the sweet potato spirals in salted boiling water for 1-2 minutes.

4 Drain the water from the pan and stir through the pesto sauce and chicken on a gentle heat for a minute or two.

5 Add the sautéed garlic and onions along with the fresh tomatoes. Combine well and serve straight away in shallow bowl.

CHEFS NOTE
Lose the chicken if you like and serve as a vegetable side.

CONVERSION CHART: DRY INGREDIENTS

Metric	Imperial
7g	¼ oz
15g	½ oz
20g	¾ oz
25g	1 oz
40g	1½oz
50g	2oz
60g	2½oz
75g	3oz
100g	3½oz
125g	4oz
140g	4½oz
150g	5oz
165g	5½oz
175g	6oz
200g	7oz
225g	8oz
250g	9oz
275g	10oz
300g	11oz
350g	12oz
375g	13oz
400g	14oz

Metric	Imperial
425g	15oz
450g	1lb
500g	1lb 2oz
550g	1¼lb
600g	1lb 5oz
650g	1lb 7oz
675g	1½lb
700g	1lb 9oz
750g	1lb 11oz
800g	1¾lb
900g	2lb
1kg	2¼lb
1.1kg	2½lb
1.25kg	2¾lb
1.35kg	3lb
1.5kg	3lb 6oz
1.8kg	4lb
2kg	4½lb
2.25kg	5lb
2.5kg	5½lb
2.75kg	6lb

CONVERSION CHART: LIQUID MEASURES

Metric	Imperial	US
25ml	1fl oz	
60ml	2fl oz	¼ cup
75ml	2½ fl oz	
100ml	3½fl oz	
120ml	4fl oz	½ cup
150ml	5fl oz	
175ml	6fl oz	
200ml	7fl oz	
250ml	8½ fl oz	1 cup
300ml	10½ fl oz	
360ml	12½ fl oz	
400ml	14fl oz	
450ml	15½ fl oz	
600ml	1 pint	
750ml	1¼ pint	3 cups
1 litre	1½ pints	4 cups

🍎 CookNation

Other COOKNATION TITLES

If you enjoyed 'The Skinny Spiralizer Recipe Book' we'd really appreciate your feedback. Reviews help others decide if this is the right book for them so a moment of your time would be appreciated.

Thank you.

You may also be interested in other '**Skinny**' titles in the CookNation series. You can find all the following great titles by searching under '**CookNation**'.

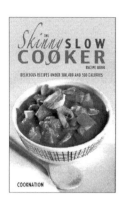

THE SKINNY SLOW COOKER RECIPE BOOK

Delicious Recipes Under 300, 400 And 500 Calories.

Paperback / eBook

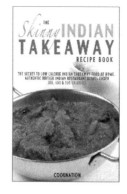

THE SKINNY INDIAN TAKEAWAY RECIPE BOOK

Authentic British Indian Restaurant Dishes Under 300, 400 And 500 Calories. The Secret To Low Calorie Indian Takeaway Food At Home.

Paperback / eBook

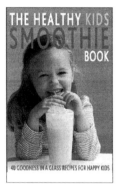

THE HEALTHY KIDS SMOOTHIE BOOK

40 Delicious Goodness In A Glass Recipes for Happy Kids.

eBook

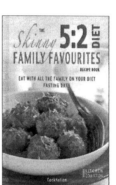

THE SKINNY 5:2 FAST DIET FAMILY FAVOURITES RECIPE BOOK

Eat With All The Family On Your Diet Fasting Days.

Paperback / eBook

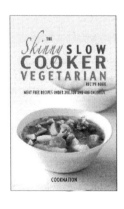

THE SKINNY SLOW COOKER VEGETARIAN RECIPE BOOK

40 Delicious Recipes Under 200, 300 And 400 Calories.

Paperback / eBook

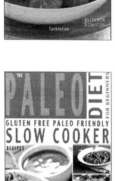

THE PALEO DIET FOR BEGINNERS SLOW COOKER RECIPE BOOK

Gluten Free, Everyday Essential Slow Cooker Paleo Recipes For Beginners.

eBook

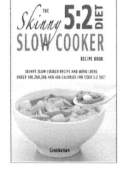

THE SKINNY 5:2 SLOW COOKER RECIPE BOOK

Skinny Slow Cooker Recipe And Menu Ideas Under 100, 200, 300 & 400 Calories For Your 5:2 Diet.

Paperback / eBook

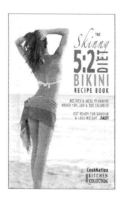

THE SKINNY 5:2 BIKINI DIET RECIPE BOOK

Recipes & Meal Planners Under 100, 200 & 300 Calories. Get Ready For Summer & Lose Weight...FAST!

Paperback / eBook

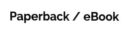

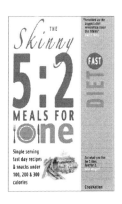

THE SKINNY 5:2 FAST DIET MEALS FOR ONE

Single Serving Fast Day Recipes & Snacks Under 100, 200 & 300 Calories.

Paperback / eBook

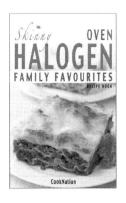

THE SKINNY HALOGEN OVEN FAMILY FAVOURITES RECIPE BOOK

Healthy, Low Calorie Family Meal-Time Halogen Oven Recipes Under 300, 400 and 500 Calories.

Paperback / eBook

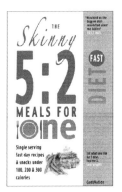

THE SKINNY 5:2 FAST DIET VEGETARIAN MEALS FOR ONE

Single Serving Fast Day Recipes & Snacks Under 100, 200 & 300 Calories.

Paperback / eBook

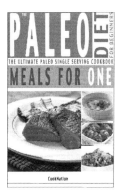

THE PALEO DIET FOR BEGINNERS MEALS FOR ONE

The Ultimate Paleo Single Serving Cookbook.

Paperback / eBook

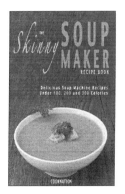

THE SKINNY SOUP MAKER RECIPE BOOK

Delicious Low Calorie, Healthy and Simple Soup Recipes Under 100, 200 and 300 Calories. Perfect For Any Diet and Weight Loss Plan.

Paperback / eBook

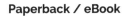

THE PALEO DIET FOR BEGINNERS HOLIDAYS

Thanksgiving, Christmas & New Year Paleo Friendly Recipes.
eBook

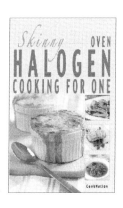

SKINNY HALOGEN OVEN COOKING FOR ONE

Single Serving, Healthy, Low Calorie Halogen Oven RecipesUnder 200, 300 and 400 Calories.

Paperback / eBook

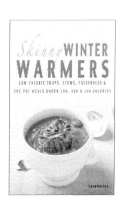

SKINNY WINTER WARMERS RECIPE BOOK

Soups, Stews, Casseroles & One Pot Meals Under 300, 400 & 500 Calories.

Paperback / eBook

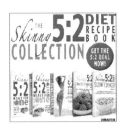

THE SKINNY 5:2 DIET RECIPE BOOK COLLECTION

All The 5:2 Fast Diet Recipes You'll Ever Need. All Under 100, 200, 300, 400 And 500 Calories.

eBook

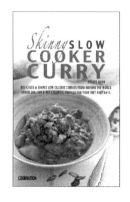

THE SKINNY SLOW COOKER CURRY RECIPE BOOK

Low Calorie Curries From Around The World.

Paperback / eBook

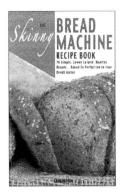

THE SKINNY BREAD MACHINE RECIPE BOOK

70 Simple, Lower Calorie, Healthy Breads...Baked To Perfection In Your Bread Maker.

Paperback / eBook

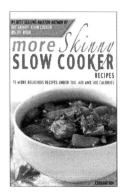

MORE SKINNY SLOW COOKER RECIPES

75 More Delicious Recipes Under 300, 400 & 500 Calories.

Paperback / eBook

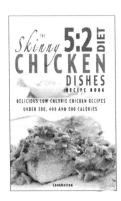

THE SKINNY 5:2 DIET CHICKEN DISHES RECIPE BOOK

Delicious Low Calorie Chicken Dishes Under 300, 400 & 500 Calories.

Paperback / eBook

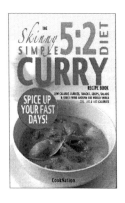

THE SKINNY 5:2 CURRY RECIPE BOOK

Spice Up Your Fast Days With Simple Low Calorie Curries, Snacks, Soups, Salads & Sides Under 200, 300 & 400 Calories.

Paperback / eBook

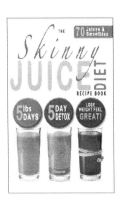

THE SKINNY JUICE DIET RECIPE BOOK

5lbs, 5 Days. The Ultimate Kick- Start Diet and Detox Plan to Lose Weight & Feel Great!

Paperback / eBook

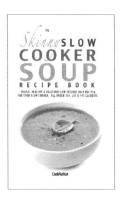

THE SKINNY SLOW COOKER SOUP RECIPE BOOK

Simple, Healthy & Delicious Low Calorie Soup Recipes For Your Slow Cooker. All Under 100, 200 & 300 Calories.

Paperback / eBook

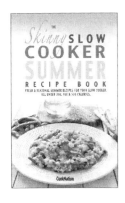

THE SKINNY SLOW COOKER SUMMER RECIPE BOOK

Fresh & Seasonal Summer Recipes For Your Slow Cooker. All Under 300, 400 And 500 Calories.

Paperback / eBook

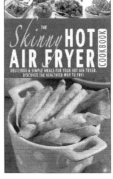

THE SKINNY HOT AIR FRYER COOKBOOK

Delicious & Simple Meals For Your Hot Air Fryer: Discover The Healthier Way To Fry.

Paperback / eBook

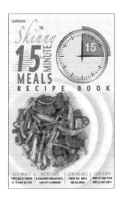

THE SKINNY ACTIFRY COOKBOOK

Guilt-free and Delicious ActiFry Recipe Ideas: Discover The Healthier Way to Fry!

Paperback / eBook

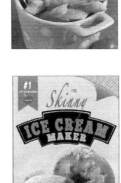

THE SKINNY ICE CREAM MAKER

Delicious Lower Fat, Lower Calorie Ice Cream, Frozen Yogurt & Sorbet Recipes For Your Ice Cream Maker.

Paperback / eBook

THE SKINNY 15 MINUTE MEALS RECIPE BOOK

Delicious, Nutritious & Super-Fast Meals in 15 Minutes Or Less. All Under 300, 400 & 500 Calories.

Paperback / eBook

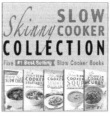

THE SKINNY SLOW COOKER COLLECTION

5 Fantastic Books of Delicious, Diet-friendly Skinny Slow Cooker Recipes: ALL Under 200, 300, 400 & 500 Calories!
eBook

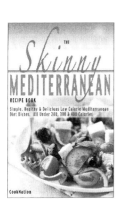

THE SKINNY MEDITERRANEAN RECIPE BOOK

Simple, Healthy & Delicious Low Calorie Mediterranean Diet Dishes. All Under 200, 300 & 400 Calories.

Paperback / eBook

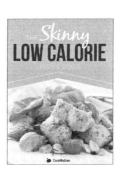

THE SKINNY LOW CALORIE RECIPE BOOK

Great Tasting, Simple & Healthy Meals Under 300, 400 & 500 Calories. Perfect For Any Calorie Controlled Diet.

Paperback / eBook

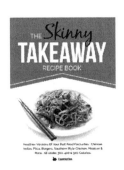

THE SKINNY TAKEAWAY RECIPE BOOK

Healthier Versions Of Your Fast Food Favourites: All Under 300, 400 & 500 Calories.

Paperback / eBook

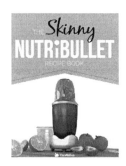

THE SKINNY NUTRIBULLET RECIPE BOOK

80+ Delicious & Nutritious Healthy Smoothie Recipes. Burn Fat, Lose Weight and Feel Great!

Paperback / eBook

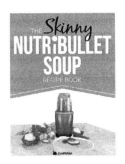

THE SKINNY NUTRIBULLET SOUP RECIPE BOOK

Delicious, Quick & Easy, Single Serving Soups & Pasta Sauces For Your Nutribullet. All Under 100, 200, 300 & 400 Calories!

Paperback / eBook

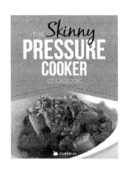

THE SKINNY PRESSURE COOKER COOKBOOK

USA ONLY
Low Calorie, Healthy & Delicious Meals, Sides & Desserts. All Under 300, 400 & 500 Calories.

Paperback / eBook

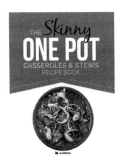

THE SKINNY ONE-POT RECIPE BOOK

Simple & Delicious, One-Pot Meals. All Under 300, 400 & 500 Calories

Paperback / eBook

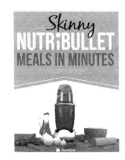

THE SKINNY NUTRIBULLET MEALS IN MINUTES RECIPE BOOK

Quick & Easy, Single Serving Suppers, Snacks, Sauces, Salad Dressings & More Using Your Nutribullet. All Under 300, 400 & 500 Calories

Paperback / eBook

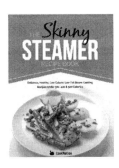

THE SKINNY STEAMER RECIPE BOOK

Healthy, Low Calorie, Low Fat Steam Cooking Recipes Under 300, 400 & 500 Calories.

Paperback / eBook

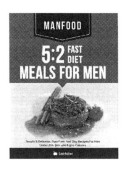

MANFOOD: 5:2 FAST DIET MEALS FOR MEN

Simple & Delicious, Fuss Free, Fast Day Recipes For Men Under 200, 300, 400 & 500 Calories.

Paperback / eBook

17460846R00054